FROM TRAU....

TO UNDERSTANDING:

A GUIDE FOR PARENTS

OF CHILDREN WITH

SEXUAL BEHAVIOR PROBLEMS

William D. Pithers

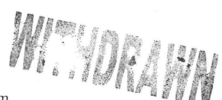

Alison S. Gray

Carolyn Cunningham

Sandy Lane

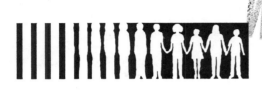

THE SAFER SOCIETY PRESS
P.O. Box 340
Brandon, VT 05733-0340
802-247-3132

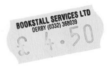

INTRODUCTION

This booklet was written for you—parents who have learned that their child has a sexual behavior problem and who want to understand and help change that behavior.

The moments following this discovery can be terribly distressing. You may begin to doubt even the most trusted relationships and question the most certain events in life. Some parents feel as if they are in a "free fall," not knowing when and how they might touch down.

Upon learning that their child has a sexual behavior problem, parents face significant decisions that influence their child's future. Even the most loving, skilled parents can feel unsure that they are making the right decisions during these moments.

This booklet offers you reassurance, guidance, and hope during a time of uncertainty. Generally, people have a hard time recalling everything they read or hear when they are feeling stressed. Thus, we encourage you to return to specific sections in this booklet for reassurance when things feel uncertain.

Preparation and publication of *From Trauma to Understanding: A Guide for Parents of Children with Sexual Behavior Problems* was funded by the Florence V. Burden Foundation. We are indebted to them for their support of this booklet and their recognition that early intervention in the troubling behaviors of children is one of the best ways of preventing problems for adults and for society.

The best wishes and hopefulness of the co-authors of this booklet and the Florence V. Burden Foundation are with you and your child as you move toward understanding.

1
COMMON FEELINGS AMONG PARENTS OF CHILDREN WITH SEXUAL BEHAVIOR PROBLEMS

If you have just learned that your child has a sexual behavior problem, you may be experiencing a wide range of feelings and thoughts all at once—which can be overwhelming. You may feel angry at your child for hurting someone, angry at yourself for having been unable to prevent it, angry at the victim or victim's family for telling, or angry at life in general. You may fear what could happen to your child and your family. Many parents feel guilty, thinking they've failed. Some parents feel embarrassed when they think about others discovering their child's problem. Other parents feel alone and ashamed, thinking that no one will understand or accept their family again. Still others find that their feelings seem numb. Some parents have all these feelings.

Many parents also may experience intense thoughts, interrupting their concentration on other tasks. You may be preoccupied with questions like, "Why did my child do that?," "Could this really have happened?," or "Did I do something wrong?" If you have not yet been able to accept that your child has a problem, you may be thinking, "Not my child!," "Boys will be boys," or "It's nobody's business what happens in my family."

If you have accepted that your child has a problem, having these questions and feelings shows that you are working to come to terms with your child's behaviors. As you do this work, you will begin to gain a sense of perspective and understanding. However, the journey toward understanding takes patience, time, and persistent effort.

Your journey toward understanding may include experiences faced by people who suffer a major loss. People recovering from major losses often pass through five stages: *Denial, Anger, Bargaining, Depression,* and *Acceptance.* These stages may be experienced one-by-one or several at once. Often, people feel that they have finished one stage, only to encounter an unexpected memory or event that takes them back to an earlier stage. These frustrating moments are really a *natural* part of the journey from trauma to understanding. Few lessons are learned perfectly the first time. If you endure, acceptance and understanding will come.

The First Stage is Denial.

In this stage, you want to believe the incident could not have happened or, if it did, that it really isn't a problem. You may think, "My child couldn't have done anything like that." You may downplay the importance of the problem and think, "They're making a big deal over nothing," or "It was only child's play."

Denial exists because we want life to stay the same as we have known it. Acknowledging a traumatic or difficult event requires us to change how we view parts of life. Again, this takes work. Denial allows us to avoid this work and to view life as we always have. Though denial is a natural first response to troubling news, we cannot deal effectively with a problem while denying that the problem exists.

The Second Stage is Anger.

People enter this stage as they become aware that a problem really exists. Anger takes many forms. You may feel angry at one person or everyone in the world. You may feel angry at your child, yourself, or the victim and his/her family. You may blame yourself, thinking, "If I had just stayed home more, this wouldn't have happened." You may hear yourself sounding like you're trying to find someone to blame for the problem, "This wouldn't have happened if they'd kept their daughter away from my son."

Anger is another step toward accepting the existence of a problem. Using anger to blame others, however, usually makes things worse, blocking our ability to look inside ourselves for things that we can do to change the situation. Rather than blaming someone, we are more effective if we find the real problems and work on them.

The Third Stage is Bargaining.

Bargaining means that people try to solve a problem by making a "deal." People often bargain when their safety seems in danger. At such moments, some people may attempt to bargain directly with God, "Let me live through this and I promise to go to church *every Sunday* for the rest of my life." While the promises are heartfelt at the moment, bargains usually are difficult to keep once the crisis has passed.

While bargaining you may have thoughts such as, "Okay, if my child goes to treatment a few times, we can just go on with our lives," "If I just spend 10 more minutes with my child every day, she'll never do that again," or "If I spend more quality time with my child he'll change these behaviors."

Bargaining occurs as we realize a problem is serious and that significant work may be needed to address it. Our "bargain" attempts to reduce the amount of work we need to do to solve the problem, the amount of emotional pain we experience, or the amount of change we need to make.

Sometimes, we actually may believe that we can bargain the problem away. However, over time, we recognize that bargaining won't take care of the problem, and work is needed.

The Fourth Stage is Depression.

Depression sets in as one realizes bargaining has not worked. Depression may leave you feeling helpless, hopeless, and sad. The reality of your child's behavior begins to sink in. If your child has been abused, you may feel even more sad.

Depression can be the hardest stage to deal with, since the lack of hope can rob your energy. However, this is a very important stage since it is a sign that you have acknowledged your child's problem and are preparing to deal with it. In this manner, the stage of depression can be seen as a temporary, intermittent period during which you are recharging your emotional battery in preparation for the work you are about to do. As depression lifts, it gives birth to hope.

The Fifth Stage is Acceptance.

Acceptance means that you can acknowledge that a problem exists. You accept that your child has hurt another child. You recognize that this problem has affected your family, that blaming outside influences for the problem will not help you find the answers, that the problem will not disappear magically, and that its solution may take work for a long period of time.

You are prepared to do the work that will help your child and family. You may feel uncertain about how the work will turn out, but you are willing to devote yourself to the effort. In reaching the stage of acceptance, you already have begun to help your child and family.

Supportive Counseling

Supportive counseling with a trained mental health professional can help you move through these stages.

Without counseling, there is a tendency to get stuck in one stage or another. Getting stuck can have negative effects for your family's recovery. If you get stuck in anger, you may feel intensely angry all of the time, blame others for your situation, or allow your anger to affect your health. If you get stuck in depression, you may become incredibly sad, losing hope that your child's behaviors can change.

Getting stuck slows down the healing process. Counseling will support you through all the stages and enable your family to make the fastest progress.

The feelings and thoughts that you are experiencing and the stages that you are going through are difficult moments in a family's life. While you may, at times, feel all alone with this problem, you are not alone. This booklet was written because thousands of parents have learned that their children have similar problems.

Many families have healed, *you and your family can heal*. By reading this booklet, you are taking an important step in understanding and dealing with your child's sexual behavior problem.

2
MYTHS AND FACTS

In the same way that our parenting skills are based primarily on the experiences we had in our own families as children, our views about sexuality are shaped by our early experiences and culture. Since our culture discourages talking openly about sexuality, all of us carry some misconceptions about it. These myths affect our behaviors, including our ability to talk about sexuality with our children.

Most of us have little information about the sexual behaviors that might be expected from a child. That's right—children normally engage in some sexual behaviors. The belief that children do not experience sexual feelings and do not engage in *any* sexual behaviors is a commonly held myth. Children experience sexual feelings and, like the rest of us, sometimes act on those feelings.

Since our beliefs affect our behaviors, let's take time to check our myths. The following list contains some common myths.

Myth: Young children do not perform sexually abusive behaviors. They are just curious.

Fact: Children *are* naturally curious about sexual information. However, children who use intimidation, verbal coercion, or force during sexual behaviors are not engaging in normal behaviors. These are signs of a sexual behavior problem.

Myth: A child with a sexual behavior problem has to have been sexually abused.

Fact: Many pathways can lead to sexual behavior problems. Some children with these problems have been abused, others have not. Younger children frequently have been sexually touched, exposed to graphic sexual information, or influenced by either an overly restricted or overly exposed sexual environment. Other children are imitating behaviors they have seen. Regardless of how your child learned these behaviors, acting out sexually or aggressively is an unacceptable way for children to get their personal needs met.

Myth: Children with sexual behavior problems will grow out of it.

Fact: While some children "self-correct," no one can tell which children will. Relying on hope that your child will self-correct gambles with your child's life and others' safety. Some young children have repeatedly abused others. Many adolescent sex offenders report that they began to abuse others during childhood, stopped the behaviors for awhile in later childhood, and resumed the abuse when they felt greater sexual interest and arousal as they became teenagers. The best way to protect your child from greater problems later in life is to get treatment for the problem now.

Myth: Children exaggerate and tell "tall tales." These stories about sexual abuse aren't real.

Fact: Children depend on adults and seek their attention in a variety of ways, including "telling stories." Almost without exception, children who talk about experiencing or performing sexually abusive behaviors are not "telling stories," they are telling the truth. As parents, our challenge is to become skilled listeners for children who courageously talk about difficult issues such as sexual abuse and sexual behavior problems. Children will not tell adults what they think adults are unable or unwilling to hear. If adults respond with shock, disgust, or anger, the child will be reluctant to talk and may begin to deny that the abusive sexual behavior actually took place. Therefore, we need to prepare ourselves to calmly hear the truth from our children.

Myth: Children are too young to remember abuse or abusing.

Fact: Children's recollections are *vastly* more rich than was once believed. Children remember many things quite accurately. In the past, we did not know how to help children express their memories. Recently, trained mental health providers have found ways of helping children recall traumatic events more accurately and to express these memories so that adults can understand them. Parents can assist children's memories of trauma and loss by maintaining a compassionate detachment, expressing belief in the child and concern for how he/she is feeling while not becoming highly emotional themselves. Children often tell adults about traumatic events in bits and pieces. We need to give them time and room to feel safe about talking.

Myth: My child would never force another child to do anything. Our child doesn't get into fights and wouldn't hurt a flea. There couldn't have been any force.

Fact: Force, or coercion, takes many forms. People can use force without being violent or using a weapon. "Force" includes pressure used to overwhelm another's ability to resist. Force can be created by verbal pressure, repeated harassment, or threatening gestures. Bribes and "tricks" also can be used to pressure a child into sex. Force can result in intimidation without the use of words when one child has greater authority, size, or strength than another.

Myth: My child does exactly as I say, so you can bet this won't happen again.

Fact: While children may conform their behaviors to our expectations, their thoughts, views, and beliefs are uniquely individual. Children may behave in a way that satisfies parental expectations and at the same time experience other beliefs, feelings, and urges. When parents aren't present, a child's beliefs guide his/her behaviors. If the child harbors thoughts about abusing others, the behavior is likely to recur. Such children need help that goes beyond parental discipline.

Considerable research has gone into discovering the facts presented here. These facts can help you accept your child's need for help in dealing with a sexual behavior problem.

3
DIFFERENTIATING NORMAL AND ABNORMAL SEXUAL DEVELOPMENT

Children pass through stages of sexual development, beginning at birth and continuing through adolescence. This chapter summarizes healthy sexual development in children as it is understood presently, then provides guidelines to help you decide whether a child's sexual behavior is appropriate. The last part of this chapter addresses fears that some parents have regarding their child's behavior.

Stages of Normal Sexual Development

Ages 0-5

Children at this age have intense curiosity about nearly everything, including their bodies, and are often happier with no clothes on. Sexual self-stimulation, or masturbation, normally begins during infancy and continues throughout development as both a self-soothing and an exciting behavior.

In addition to their own bodies, children of these ages also are curious about others' bodies. Their curiosity may lead them to try to look at or touch others' genitalia. This is *exploratory* looking and touching, typically accompanied by giggling and amusement rather than *coercion*. When clear limits are set, preschoolers take redirection easily.

Ages 6-10

School-age children continue to explore their bodies. Curiosity about sexuality takes the form of playing games such as "doctor" or "I'll show you mine if you show me yours." Boys at this age compare penis size. Children become interested in sex words and dirty jokes. Limited interest in the opposite sex may be evident. Interest in their own and others' bodies continues during this time, particularly if changes in their bodies begin to occur.

Preadolescence (Ages 11-12)

Masturbation continues during preadolescence. Preadolescents are focused on establishing relationships with peers. Some preadolescents engage in sexual activity with peers, including kissing and fondling. Preadolescents may imitate sexual behaviors that they have seen or heard about. While most of these experiences are with the opposite sex, preadolescents may engage in sexual activities with their own gender. Such sexual activity with one's own gender does not necessarily indicate homosexuality. Normal sexual behaviors focus on consenting activities with peers, respecting the limits set by their partner.

Sexual Behavior Problems

How can we tell when a sexual behavior is a problem? Five criteria are used to determine whether a sexual behavior is normal or abusive: 1) whether the type of sexual activity is normally expected for the child's developmental level; 2) whether the children involved have relatively equal power; 3) whether force or intimidation was used; 4) whether the behavior is kept secret; and 5) whether the behavior appears compulsive or the child is obsessed with it.

1) Sexual Activity Compared to Developmental Level.

As a first step in deciding whether a sexual behavior is a problem, compare your child's developmental level to the *type* of sexual activity your child is performing. Is it beyond the developmental level of your child?

For example, oral-genital intercourse is beyond the behaviors expected from children under age 5. Any sexual behaviors based on threats or suggesting preoccupation with abusive sexuality also suggest that a problem exists.

Children aged 6-10 who attempt genital or anal penetration, genital kissing, or oral-genital intercourse have a sexual behavior problem.

A child, aged 10-12, who engages in sex play with much younger children, or who forces someone to engage in sex, has a sexual behavior problem.

2) Relative Power of Children.

If one child participating in a sexual activity has more power than another, it is more likely that the sexual behavior is a problem. Is one child much older than the other? If one child is 10 and the other 5, the 10 year-old has much more power than the 5 year-old. In addition to age, other factors can create differences in power. If one child has a severe learning disability and another has normal intelligence, a difference in power exists. A child who is much taller or stronger than another has greater power. Also, if one child is always the "leader" and the other is always the "follower," there is a difference in power.

3) Use of Intimidation, Force, Trickery, or Bribes.

Check whether the behavior involved intimidation, force, trickery, or bribes. If so, this suggests a sexual behavior problem. Developmentally normal sexual behaviors involve curiosity and game-playing, not intimidation, force, trickery, or bribes.

4) Secrecy.

It may be difficult to distinguish a child's natural sense of privacy or embarrassment about sexual feelings from the secrecy that allows abusive sexuality to continue. Privacy is a rightful protection from intrusion, while secrecy suggests that a child is avoiding the consequences of an action he/she knows or senses is wrong or causes harm.

5) Compulsiveness or Obsessiveness.

Does the behavior appear compulsive (seeming as if the child can't control it) or obsessional (something the child thinks about continually)? These are signs of a sexual behavior problem.

These are rough guidelines for evaluating your child's sexual behaviors. Any one of them may or may not be a sign of a problem. If you have any concerns, an evaluation of your child's behavior by a trained mental health professional can determine whether your child needs help.

Parents' Concerns
About Children with Sexual Behavior Problems

As a parent of a child with a sexual behavior problem, some of your fears might include:

1. Will my child become an adolescent or adult sex offender?

No one can say for sure that a child who acts out sexually will become an adolescent or adult offender. Some adolescent and adult offenders report that they started sexually abusing as children. If your child is acting out sexually, it is a sign that something is wrong and help is needed. Providing that help *now* is the best way of preventing problems later in life.

2. If my child was molested by someone of the same sex will my child be a homosexual?

Sexual abuse does not cause someone to be gay, lesbian, or heterosexual. Heterosexuality and homosexuality are not diseases someone "catches," they are sexual orientations. In fact, recent evidence suggests that sexual orientation is influenced by factors that take place before birth.

3. Is there something wrong if my child says that sexually acting out feels good?

Sexual arousal itself is normal and feels good. It is what the arousal is associated with that determines whether a problem exists. In adults, arousal to thoughts about sexual expression of intimacy is healthy, but arousal to thoughts about violent or coercive sex is a problem.

Sexual arousal in children creates problems when it is associated with memories of prior sexual abuse, or feelings of fear, anxiety, or anger. Your child needs help to separate the part that feels good—the arousal—from the negative feelings, situations, and behaviors that are associated with it.

In summary, sexual behavior problems are a concern if a child uses intimidation, force, trickery, or bribes; is significantly older or more powerful than the other person; or engages in developmentally inappropriate acts.

4
WHY DO CHILDREN ABUSE?

There is no single cause for childhood sexual behavior problems. Many things could be related to sexual behavior problems. A treatment professional, working with your child and family, may offer therapeutic suggestions about ways of lessening the influence of these factors.

If you were to ask your child "Why?," he or she would probably say, "I don't know." They aren't lying to you since many children, particularly younger children, don't know all the reasons they act abusively. However, treatment providers who have worked with children who abuse can identify some common causes.

Children abuse other children because it makes them feel better in some way. Sometimes it gives children a momentary sense of relief emotionally or physically. It's not a "feel good" like sex is for adults. For adults, healthy sexual activity is associated with anticipation and experience of intense physical pleasure and psychological intimacy.

For children with sexual behavior problems, the physical sensations of sex can be present, but the most powerful "feel good" occurs in their minds and emotions. Some of the thoughts and emotions associated with these behaviors include:

♦ Some children feel more popular or grown-up when they engage in sexual behaviors.

♦ Some children believe they'll feel less weak or helpless if they can persuade another child to be sexual with them.

♦ Some children feel less worried about their problems when they experience sex.

♦ Some children feel excited doing something they know adults won't like, especially if they think they won't get caught.

♦ Some children are curious about sexual behaviors they have heard about or seen.

♦ Some children have been abused and repeat behaviors that were sexually stimulating, or they may be attempting to undo or understand the behavior by repeating it.

- Some children like the way their body feels when their private parts are touched.

- Some children don't know that it's not okay to make another child do sexual behaviors.

- For some children, the behavior has become a habit; they might feel unable to stop.

- Some children think it's fun, not recognizing how their behavior affects others.

Although a child might "feel good" while abusing, it lasts for a very short time. Afterwards, they worry about getting in trouble or feel bad about what they did. Sometimes they get so worried and think about it so much, they do it again to seek relief from feeling bad. As a result, children can get into a vicious cycle of abusing.

Children tell us that the "feel good" is so strong that they will do a lot of things they wouldn't usually do to make sure they can get this feeling. They may think about which child they can get to do this behavior, usually picking one they think won't tell and won't be able to stop them. They think about ways they can trick or make the other child cooperate. They think about how and where to do it without getting caught. They think about what they can say to stay out of trouble if they are caught.

Most children feel a tug-of-war in their conscience about what they are doing. They may know what they are doing is wrong, yet enjoy the intensity of the "feel good" feeling. In order to lessen the guilt, they make up excuses about why the abusive behavior was "okay."

Children, who may not realize how much sexual abuse hurts other children, have a hard time putting themselves in another's shoes and are surprised when they are told that their sexual behavior hurt someone.

Some things can make children at risk to abuse other children. Sexual, physical, or emotional abuse, abandonment, or exposure to a sexualized environment are often present in the histories of many children with sexual behavior problems. Living in a chaotic family, feeling bad about themselves, and not knowing how others feel are also common. Lacking good social skills (such as knowing how to join in children's games or how to make friends) and not knowing how to handle uncomfortable feelings are difficulties that add to the risk of sexual behavior problems.

When a child thinks about sexual abuse, some things make it more likely that he/she will decide to go ahead and do it. These things include: "sticky thinking" or excuses that make it seem okay, situations offering an opportunity for the behavior to occur without being caught, being upset about something and not talking about it, not telling themselves that abusive behavior is hurtful, or having strong urges and thoughts about what they would like to do, and not being able to use self-control.

Once children start sexually abusing, some things increase the potential that they will do it again. These include the memory of the powerful "feel good" feelings experienced during abuse, not understanding what sexual behaviors are not okay, not being told that their behavior is not okay, being left alone in situations where they have power over another child, not taking responsibility for what they have done and blaming others, feeling ashamed or bad about themselves, and not having someone to talk to about their feelings.

5
WHAT HAPPENS IN TREATMENT?

Supportive counseling is an essential part of your child's and your family's healing and recovery. People who aren't familiar with what happens in counseling may be reluctant to enter treatment because they fear this unknown process.

Counseling takes place in a very private setting. Your child and you may each be seen alone (individual therapy), with others (group treatment), or together as family (family therapy). You could be involved in a combination of these treatments. Treatment sessions may occur once, twice, or sometimes three times a week. The frequency of your sessions depends on the types of treatment you are receiving and how many sessions your counselor feels would help.

A counselor has received professional training in ways to support your family and child, and can help you understand your child's behaviors.

If you find it difficult to develop trust with your counselor, you are free to change until you find one you can trust. Just as you choose the right doctor for your health problems, you can choose the right counselor for your family and child.

The types of questions people ask when they begin treatment include:

1. Won't this problem go away by itself?

The answer is most likely "no." It is important to understand that your child's behavior is a sign that something is going on that is upsetting or confusing. Without getting to the root of the problem, it is difficult to decrease or change the problem behavior.

The behavior may appear to stop for awhile even if your child does not complete treatment, but the basic problems that motivated your child's behaviors will remain. Therefore, without treatment, the behavior most likely will recur in the future. It resembles a splinter in your finger. Even if you can't see the splinter, you can feel it irritating you until it is taken out.

If something is upsetting your child, your child will continue to act out or feel upset until the problem is resolved.

2. My family's problems are private. No one outside my family needs to know about them.

There is no escaping the fact that sexual behavior problems are difficult to discuss. However, open discussion of these problems in a therapeutic setting is essential to your child's and family's recovery. Such discussions break the secrecy that allows sexual abuse to continue. By openly discussing these problems during treatment, you might gain new ideas you can use to stop your child's problem behaviors.

Counselors are required by law and professional ethics to keep your conversations private. This is called "confidentiality." You have the right to confidentiality within counseling sessions, even if the sessions involve other people in a group setting. Only a few exceptions to confidentiality exist. If you sign a "waiver of confidentiality" form, you give your therapist permission to talk to the person whose name is shown on the form. If your child reveals having abused another child, your counselor is legally required to inform child protective services so that the other child can receive help. Similarly, the therapist is required by law to report to authorities any child abuse you may have performed. Finally, if your child appears to represent a clear and present danger to his/her own safety or the safety of someone else, (for instance, by making threats of suicide or threats against the victim), the therapist may be required to break confidentiality so that your child can receive more help. If you have any questions about confidentiality, ask your counselor.

Most parents need help dealing with their child's sexual behavior problems. Counselors will help your family work through this problem. They are trained to support you and help your child control his/her behavior, not to invade your privacy.

3. If I pray hard enough, and get support through my church, isn't that enough?

Your church, synagogue, mosque, and any other community sources of support available to you are important for your child's and family's recovery. They can give you spiritual and inner strength during moments when you question your ability to hang in there.

Ultimately, you must discover your own course, steer your own recovery, and help steer the recovery of your child. Your mental health counselor is specially trained to help your child and family understand sexual behavior problems, and can be an important source of therapeutic and emotional support.

4. Why do I need to go to therapy? My child is the one with the problem!

Your child needs support and encouragement. You are *the most important support person to your child.* You can assist your child's efforts to change by understanding your child's patterns and helping your child control them. You are a part of your child's "safety team;" without your support, the chances of your child abusing again are increased.

In addition, if you have been sexually abused, or if you are experiencing other stresses, your child's behaviors may bring up memories and feelings that make it difficult for you to address your child's problem. If this is true for you, counseling may help you with these stresses, helping you to feel better, and enabling you to deal more effectively with your child's needs.

5. I don't have enough money to come every week, but I can make it once in a while.

In order for treatment to be effective, your attendance and your child's must be regular and consistent. Attending treatment once in a while will not work. Particularly when a child has obsessive thoughts about abusive behaviors, treatment needs to be consistent. Many mental health centers have sliding fee scales to assist you with the financial issues.

6. I have been a good parent. I don't understand where my child got this behavior. I can take this into my own hands.

The fact that your child has a problem does not mean you are a bad parent. It means that your child needs help and understanding. Taking things into your own hands, alone, is not a good idea. Everyone needs help sometimes. Right now, specialized treatment is the help needed for your child's healthy development. Going into treatment may be difficult at first, but most people find it supportive and are glad they did it.

First Visits

The first few times you go to a counselor, you may be asked to complete an *assessment.* This assessment is done in order to quickly find out as much as possible about factors that may play a role in your child's problem. The assessment phase may involve two different kinds of information-gathering: 1) interviews with your child and you and 2) paper-and-pencil tests.

Throughout counseling, neither you nor your child should be blamed or scolded. The counselor will talk to you to learn your child's history, any problems your child has had, how your child handles different feelings, and what you know about your child's sexual behavior. It is always very helpful if you can describe all the things that you have noticed that your child has said or done that might let the counselor know more about your child.

The counselor also will talk with your child, asking questions about your child's feelings, thoughts, and sexual behaviors. Depending on your child's age, the interview may involve talking while your child plays, or just sitting and talking. The questions will be very specific because that usually makes a child feel more comfortable and understood. If your child is having trouble admitting he/she has a sexual behavior problem, the treatment person will try to help your child feel okay about getting out feelings of denial, anger, or depression.

You and your child may be asked to take some tests to get more information about your child's life. The tests don't have "right" or "wrong" answers. Some tests might ask you to check off behaviors that your child shows, some might ask you to rate how often you or your child experience certain emotions or thoughts, others might request short written answers to questions, and some might have either of you draw pictures.

After the initial assessment is completed, the treatment provider should be willing to tell you what he or she has learned about your child.

Your counselor may ask you and/or your child to complete the assessment again after you have been in therapy awhile. This is done in order to insure that treatment is following the right course.

Treatment Groups

Your child may take part in group treatment with other children. Group treatment seems to help children in a different way than individual therapy. In group treatment, children learn they are not the only person with this problem and, as a result, they begin to feel better about themselves. Sometimes it is easier for a child to understand when they hear other children describing how they think and feel. Some elements of the group treatment focus on general topics that help all children who abuse children and some may address issues unique to your child.

Younger children can only pay attention for a short time. Therefore, the treatment group may be divided into sections. The children will have a time to share things that have happened since the last meeting, a time to learn a new idea that helps them control their behavior, a time to practice new skills, and a time for closing the group. There may be a time for structured play or for parents to join their children as the session ends.

There probably will be some homework for both you and your child. After each session, you may meet with the counselor to learn what your child is working on or in a parents' treatment group at the same time that your child's group is meeting. You may be asked to observe your child for some type of behavior during the next week, to remind your child of something he/she is trying to practice, or to help your child learn a new habit.

The counselor will try to work closely with you so that you can help your child gain control of his/her behavior. It will be important for the counselor to know what problems your child has when he/she is not in group to lessen the chances of your child engaging in another harmful behavior. When you, your child, and your child's treatment provider combine your efforts to control your child's problem behavior, you become the *Prevention Team*. As teammates, you work together toward a common goal: a healthy, thriving child who lives free from the destructiveness of a sexual behavior problem.

Treatment Goals

Treatment helps your child learn to control his/her abusive behavior. There is no easy "cure" that will make the problem go away, but many children have learned to stop the behavior from happening again. Another goal is to provide your child with skills that may make the urges less frequent because he/she has learned to "feel good" in appropriate ways. Your child also will learn new ways to handle feelings that may contribute to his/her problem.

Some of the general goals that your child will work on include:

◆ Admitting he/she has a problem with sexual behavior.

◆ Understanding the steps or patterns your child goes through each time he/she sexually abuses.

- Developing ways to interrupt each step in your child's pattern.

- Eliminating "sticky thinking" that helps your child believe the behavior is okay.

- Working with past traumas or losses.

- Developing better self-control to prevent your child from repeating the abusive behavior.

- Learning skills that can help your child handle problems and "feel good" in non-hurtful ways.

- Understanding how your child's behavior made the other child and his/her own family feel.

- Learning what situations are risky and how to handle or avoid them.

- Asking for assistance from others during times when your child doubts his/her self-control.

- Increasing your child's skill at perspective-taking and moral reasoning.

You may be asked to provide supervision in a way that helps your child use what he/she is learning and helps your child to control his/her behavior in the future. Your participation is critical since your family's therapist may work only 1 hour a week with your child. If you provide your child with effective supervision during the remaining hours of the week, your child's progress through treatment will benefit greatly. Together, you and your therapist can work as an effective team, offering assistance to your child.

Roadblocks to Progress in Treatment

To help children, parents need to possess accurate information, see a wide range of choices, make decisions carefully, act confrontively when necessary, persist during difficult moments, and reward progress. Since children learn by watching their parents, being careful to control your own behaviors will assist your child.

Parents can model a willingness to examine and change their own thoughts and behaviors, replacing quick assumptions with careful consideration. For example, when we have problems at work, our quick assumption may be that our boss is being unfair. This would allow us to view someone else as the source of our problem. We would be using "sticky thinking," sticking someone else with responsibility for a problem, in this case "blaming" our boss.

While sticky thinking helps us feel better or righteously indignant, it does not contribute to constructive solutions to problems. It allows us to feel angry at someone else rather than disappointed in ourselves. Sticky thinking also can be used to excuse or justify our behaviors ("You made me lie to you."). Children with sexual behavior problems may use sticky thinking in order to excuse their abuse of another child ("I only wanted to make him feel good."). In treatment, children learn how to identify and change sticky thinking in order to solve the problems they face.

We all occasionally slide responsibility away from ourselves when we are uncomfortable with something we did, said, or neglected to do. However, frequent use of sticky thinking by parents is not helpful to children. It is important for you to try to change sticky thinking, such as blaming, excuse-making, lying by leaving something out, or justifying. You can do this by practicing four steps: **Catch, Stop, Replace,** and **Review.**

Catch your sticky thinking by noticing statements that start with words like "But..., I can't..., You should..., You always..., I only..., I never...". Practice with a partner giving your own examples. What is your most frequent sticky thought? Watch for its appearance as you talk with relatives, your child, or family. Be on guard for its appearance when you feel anxious, angry, or defensive. Sticky thoughts might emerge as you think about entering treatment.

The following list was created by parents who were involved in treatment with their children and suggests some types of sticky thoughts you might watch for:

1) I don't have time to take part in my child's treatment.

2) I don't think I should have to attend treatment, I didn't do anything wrong.

3) Treatment doesn't work. It only makes things worse.

4) This whole process is abusive to my child and family.

5) I am the real victim here.

6) If there is no injury there is no harm done.

7) My children are my property. They'll do what I tell them.

8) The victim asked for it.

9) They were just playing. You mean children can't be curious anymore?

10) They were only playing doctor. It didn't mean anything.

11) I did that when I was a child and I'm okay. My child will be okay too.

Removing Roadblocks:

Overcoming sticky thinking with confrontive thinking opens doors instead of closes doors. Confrontive thinking enables you to create solutions. You are a strong role model for your child when you interrupt your own sticky thinking. You give your child an example to learn from, while gaining benefits for yourself as well.

After you **catch** the thought and **stop** it from taking on a life of its own, you can **replace** the sticky thought with one that is more helpful to you and your child. Below is a list of constructive responses for some of the sticky thoughts listed earlier:

1) My time is valuable. If I invest it now, I may prevent my time being disrupted later and also may prevent another victimization.

2) If I take part in treatment, I will learn how to help my child at home. If I do this, my child may be able to make faster progress. It's one way of showing my concern for my child's health.

3) Sometimes things seem to get worse after a treatment session. Maybe it's like going to the dentist. Fixing a tooth is sometimes painful. After the pain goes away, the tooth is healthier than ever.

4) This has been disruptive to our family, and the family and I
& are victims, too. However, we will end the disruption by
5) working to make things better. If I let myself get furious about this, I may contribute to my child's problem.

6) Sometimes the biggest problems in life are the least visible. Even though the victim doesn't seem different on the outside, I cannot judge how much she/he was really harmed.

7) I will pay greater attention to my own behavior, as well as my child's. However, I do not have the ability to "control" my child. I recognize the limits of my control. The only person I can control is myself.

8) I don't think my child intended to harm anyone. Yet, my
to child's behavior has harmed the other child. I need to do what
11) I can to support my child's efforts not to hurt someone else.

After you successfully *catch, stop,* and *replace* a sticky thought, take time to *review* how well your replacement thoughts worked. Do you feel more sure about the steps to take to help your child? Are your thoughts less angry? Do you have a sense of perspective on your child's behaviors and your responses? Even though you may not see the end of the road, can you see that you are on the road? If so, these are signs that you have done a good job of interrupting and replacing your sticky thinking. If not, use some new thoughts to *replace* the old ones, then *review* again.

This four-step process may not work "perfectly" the first time. Most people usually don't get things "perfectly right" on their first try. While no amount of practice ever makes one perfect, you'll find that practice can make you "good enough" to change your sticky thoughts.

6
CARING FOR YOURSELF

Concerned parents sometimes devote so much attention to their children that they neglect to take care of their own needs. This tendency can be strongest when children have problems. During such times, it is possible to get to the point where we feel guilty taking any time away from our children in order to meet our own needs. No matter how much we love our children, if we totally neglect our own needs, our self-neglect will interfere with our ability to function as good parents.

As you demonstrate self-caring behaviors, your child learns to do the same (from your example), and both of you will have more energy to deal with stresses and challenges. If you are tired, exhausted, stressed and strained, worried and feeling overwhelmed or scared, angry or helpless, it is all the more important for you to increase your efforts to attend to your emotional needs. Again, doing so will give you energy, and provide a good "I take care of myself" model for your child. Children learn by watching more than by listening.

By taking care of ourselves, our thoughts, and our feelings, we provide healthy models for children. This process is called self-care, very different from being selfish. Self-care is taking responsibility for meeting our own emotional, physical, and psychological needs without neglecting others' needs. Selfishness is defined by *consistently* caring *only* about one's *own* needs. Self-caring parents work to meet their own needs, just as they work to meet the emotional, physical, and psychological needs of their children.

What ways do you already demonstrate self-care? List some now. This might be a difficult task because you may be so busy that thinking of taking care of yourself seems foreign or silly to you, or you might live in an area where escape from everyday stresses seems impossible. Changing this pattern may take some work. Identifying self-caring behaviors that you see in others may be helpful. Giving yourself permission to develop a self-care plan is a first step. Some ways parents have started this process include:

- Taking a hot bath for relaxation.

- Taking a walk or jogging once a day.

- Regularly calling a friend just to talk—and not only about the crisis situation.

- Finding a quiet spot and listening to silence.
- Reading for fun.
- Planning a regular time for exercise.

Be sure to make your plan realistic. Find someone with whom you can share your self-care successes. If you *occasionally* do not stick to your plan, don't condemn yourself. If you *consistently* do not live up to your plan, examine and revise it. One way of undermining your effort is to create a very unrealistic plan, be unable to stick to it, and feel like a failure. So be realistic as you set and revise your self-care plans.

By taking even a few minutes a day for yourself, you increase your ability to be a resourceful, responsible parent. Start right now by selecting one thing you will do for yourself today that is kind and nurturing to you. Start with something small. Give yourself permission to do it and be prepared to ask for the support you may need to establish a new self-care pattern.

If You Are An Abuse Survivor

Estimates suggest that 1 in 4 females and at least 1 in 9 males in our society have been sexually abused; many more people have been physically or emotionally abused. If you have been abused, your child's behaviors may have reawakened painful memories for you. If so, the emotions you experienced upon learning of your child's abusiveness may feel extreme and out-of-control, making it more difficult, at least temporarily, to address your child's behaviors.

Self-examination requires courage. All of us are reluctant to make ourselves vulnerable to painful memories and emotions without a good reason. Dealing with past influences shows great concern for your child and yourself. Let us not expect our children to be the first to handle the tough issues. Let us not ask them to make a trek through recovery alone. To serve as guides for our children, we need to be willing to take the journey ourselves first.

If you choose to seek counseling for your own abuse, you do not need to be alone. Specialized counselors and support groups can help you. Working with others who have experienced abuse often helps greatly. Parents who have entered treatment to address their own abuse tell us that it was a hard decision to make, but one they recommend to other parents because of the support and success they experienced.

If you are curious about what support is out there for you, research your options just as you would before making any important decision. Ask questions before agreeing to work with a counselor or group on an ongoing basis. You need to feel a high degree of trust in your counselor in order to benefit as much as possible. Remember that strength grows from practice and improvement. You can demonstrate this lesson for your children.

If You or Your Partner Have Abused Your Child

If you or your partner has abused your child emotionally, physically, or sexually, it may be necessary for the abuser to step out of a parental role for the time being. Children may not feel safe when around someone who has abused them. Your child may not be able to tell the abuser this directly. Your child may be afraid of being hurt again by telling you how he/she really feels.

If you are the abuser, you may be asked to leave your home for a period of time and to take part in a treatment group for abusers. You will benefit from this by learning how to interrupt your own abusive pattern and your child will benefit since he/she can remain at home, feeling safe and supported by your spouse and any other children in your family. You may be asked not to have any contact with your child or you may be permitted to visit your child only when a responsible adult, who can monitor your visit, is present.

By accepting these conditions and, in specialized treatment, working to change your hurtful behavior, you can begin to restore others' faith in your concern for your child and your ability to control your behaviors. You may feel uncomfortable about this process, but it will increase your child's comfort and your accountability for your own behaviors. You will give your child a better chance at recovering from the abuse.

7
DEALING WITH AGENCIES, THERAPISTS, AND THE PREVENTION TEAM

Parents have told us that some of the most difficult moments in the journey from trauma to understanding have involved tense interactions with representatives of state agencies or departments that are involved with their family.

Information is power. Ask questions! Be an educated consumer who learns about resources the system can contribute to help your child.

You do not have to be the expert or have all the answers. In regard to sexual behavior problems of childhood, there are no "experts." No one possesses all the answers. Everyone can offer some help in solving problems.

Keep in mind you are most effective when you create a way to examine each uncomfortable piece of this puzzle. Look out for sticky thoughts that encourage you to create disputes where none need exist. Model your behaviors after those of parents who demonstrate victim empathy, self-accountability, and a willingness to work with the system to gain access to resources for the benefit of their children.

Nothing in life is truly "perfect." These systems are not perfect, nor are the people working in them. Their goals are generally to protect public safety and to help your child not repeat the abusive behavior. Often there are legal or budgetary restrictions that limit what agency workers can do to help. And sometimes the most caring worker can have a bad day like the rest of us.

Try to problem-solve with the worker first.

Get as much information as possible.

If the problem persists, ask a supervisor to explain the course of action that is in dispute.

Ask for the opportunity to correct any possible misinformation on which a decision might be based.

Especially in moments of dispute, remember to let your integrity lead you.

8
HOME-BASED INTERVENTIONS

Most children have some ability to use self-control, but they are still learning. They need supervision and help. You are in the best position to provide help, but if others sometimes care for your child, you need to teach them how to supervise your child. There are some clear procedures and steps you can put into place that can have a *tremendous* impact on your child's self-management and safety. Among these steps are: 1) decreasing opportunity to abuse, 2) teaching sexual safety and privacy rules, 3) encouraging open communications, 4) limiting experiences that increase sexual thoughts, 5) interrupting and redirecting misuse of power, 6) correcting sticky thinking, and 7) staying calm. Here are some examples of these simple steps:

Decrease Opportunity

- Don't leave your child alone with victim-age children.

- Don't have your child and a known victim bathe, sleep, or change clothes together.

- If your child is playing with another child, stay in the room or check on them frequently.

- Discourage games your child may have used to get another child to go along with the sexual behavior (playing doctor, house, Simon Says, hide-and-go-seek, freeze the statue, etc.).

Teach Sexual Safety and Privacy Rules

- Bathrooms are private; others don't enter when someone is bathing or using the toilet.

- Doors are closed when someone is changing or using a bathroom.

- Bedrooms are private; other children enter only with an adult.

- Clothing is worn when one is in the presence of others.

- One should knock and wait for permission before opening a closed door.

Encourage Open Communication

+ Listen to your child when he/she shares feelings, problems or worries—compliment your child for sharing.

+ Help your child figure out what to do about his/her worries. Avoid just saying "Don't worry" or "It'll be okay."

+ Give your child permission to share both negative and positive feelings.

Limit Experiences That Increase Sex Thoughts

+ Don't expose your child to movies, soap operas, or music that show sexual or violent themes.

+ Interrupt sexual jokes, stories, and language and describe how this can harm others.

+ When adults engage in sexual behaviors, they should do so in private settings where they cannot be observed.

+ Talk with your children about their sexual concerns and give clear, consistent messages about what is and is not okay.

+ Give clear messages about when and where masturbation or touching one's own private parts is okay and having healthy, nonabusive thoughts while doing this.

+ Videos and magazines containing graphic violence or sex should not be stored or used by adults at home.

Interrupt and Redirect Misuse of Power

+ Discourage your child's bossiness or use of force to handle problems with another child. Help them problem-solve other ways to handle each situation.

+ Encourage your child to feel good about his/her efforts. Discourage the belief that your child has to be best, the first, or have the most to be okay.

+ Help your child say what he/she is feeling during acting out behavior. Help your child think about other ways to handle those feelings.

+ Set limits and give clear messages that it is not okay to hurt someone else.

Correct Sticky Thinking

◆ When you hear your child say something that supports his/her sexual behavior problem, help your child to replace it with a corrected thought (such as replacing "I can do what I want" with "No, some things aren't safe, I have to follow some rules").

◆ Interrupt thoughts that allow your child to view him- or herself as being "victimized" by your discipline (such as, "You don't love me because you said no" with "I do love you; I don't want you to do this because...").

◆ Remind your child how others feel or are affected by his/her behaviors.

◆ Help your child say how he/she feels or is affected by problems that he/she experiences.

Stay Calm

◆ Help your child feel he/she can tell you about what occurred. You can let your child know you don't approve but want to help him/her not do it again.

◆ Let your child know that you want to hear when he/she is having sexual thoughts so you can help your child control the problem behaviors.

◆ If you observe your child starting to engage in a sexually abusive behavior, calmly interrupt it, state why it is not okay, and help your child figure out how he/she can stop it or control it—stay with your child to provide control.

◆ If your child repeats a behavior, let him/her know it is not okay but that you still want to work together to not let it happen again—know that your child may slip and it's a hard behavior to interrupt because it "feels good."

We hope this booklet has offered you a source of hope. Hope is a precious resource essential to recovery. During the moments you feel down, recall that depression gives birth to hope. Persistence is necessary during the journey from trauma to understanding. Difficulties encountered during this journey are made easier if you are willing to travel with companions. Trust your family, your counselor, or a support group to be traveling companions who want to hear your concerns when difficult moments occur. Trust their ability to carry some of your burden. Trust that, with effort, you will reach your destination. Its name is Understanding.